Mediterranean Diet

Mediterranean Diet Recipes & Desserts You Can Cook At Home

(Lose Weight In 7 Days With Easy, Delicious Meals)

Ernest Valentine

Published by Jason Thawne Publishing House

© Ernest Valentine

Mediterranean Diet: Mediterranean Diet Recipes & Desserts You Can Cook At Home (Lose Weight in 7 Days With Easy, Delicious Meals)

All Rights Reserved

ISBN 978-1-989749-92-0

This document is geared towards providing exact and reliable information in regards to the topic and issue covered. The publication is sold with the idea that the publisher isn't required to render accounting, officially permitted, or otherwise, qualified services. If advice is necessary, legal or even professional, a practiced individual in the profession should be ordered.

- From a Declaration of Principles which was accepted and approved equally by a Committee of the American Bar Association and a Committee of Publishers and Associations.

In no way is it legal to reproduce, duplicate, or even transmit any part of this document in either electronic means or in printed format. Recording of this publication is strictly prohibited and any storage of this document isn't allowed unless with proper written permission from the publisher. All rights reserved.

The information provided herein is stated to be truthful and consistent, in that any liability, in terms of inattention or otherwise, by any usage or abuse of any policies, processes, or directions contained within is the solitary and also utter responsibility of the recipient reader. Under no circumstances will any legal responsibility or blame be held against the publisher for any reparation, damages, or monetary loss due to the information herein, either directly or indirectly.

Respective authors own all copyrights not held by the publisher.

The information herein is offered for just informational purposes solely, and is universal as so. The presentation of the information is without contract or any type of guarantee assurance.

The trademarks that are used are without any consent, and also the publication of the trademark is without permission or backing by the trademark owner. All trademarks and brands within this book are for clarifying purposes only and are the owned by the owners themselves, not affiliated with this document.

TABLE OF CONTENTS

PART 1 1

INTRODUCTION 2

CHAPTER 1: KNOW THE MEDITERRANEAN DIET 4

CHAPTER 2: THE BASICS OF A MEDITERRANEAN DIET 12

CHAPTER 3: PLANNING A MEDITERRANEAN DIET 24

CHAPTER 4: 7-DAY MEDITERRANEAN MEAL PLAN 34

DAY-4 38

DAY-5 38

CHAPTER 5: MEDITERRANEAN DIET RECIPES 41

SOFT AND FLUFFY PANCAKES 42

GREEK-STYLED OMELET 45

BREAKFAST COUSCOUS 46

BANANA-AND-NUT OATMEAL 47

ZUCCHINI FRITTATA WITH GOAT CHEESE 48

BERRIES-AND-YOGURT PARFAIT 50

GREEK-STYLED SALAD 51

GREEK CHICKEN SALAD WITH HERBS 52

PASTA SALAD 54

PANZANELLA 56

WHITE BEAN SOUP 57

GRILLED VEGETABLE TAGINE 59

GRILLED EGGPLANT SANDWICH 61

MEDITERRANEAN-STYLE FISH FILLET 63

DINNER SALAD... 64

STUFFED TOMATOES 66

CHICKPEA PATTIES 67

CHICKEN THIGHS STUFFED WITH TOMATO SAUCE............ 69

GREEK PIZZA 72

OLIVES-IN-HERBS 74

ROASTED CHICKPEAS 74

CREAM-COVERED BLUEBERRIES 75

TOMATO SKEWERS 76

POACHED PEARS.. 77

MARINATED OLIVES WITH FETA 79

MEDITERRANEAN RICE PUDDING 80

CONCLUSION 82

PART 2 84

INTRODUCTION 85

WHAT IS A MEDITERRANEAN DIET 85

WHAT FOODS ARE INCLUDED IN THE MEDITERRANEAN DIET 92

WHAT ARE THE HEALTH BENEFITS OF THE MEDITERRANEAN DIET... 110

HOW TO LOSE WEIGHT ON THE MEDITERRANEAN DIET . 111

IMPLEMENTING A MEDITERRANEAN DIET PLAN............. 111

SAMPLE MEAL PLAN 112

RECIPE 113

CONCLUSION ....**ERROR! BOOKMARK NOT DEFINED.**

Part 1

Introduction

Diets have become a regular part of our lives, whether we want it to be or not. Every day, we hear and see thousands of new information everyday telling us to eat this, and not to eat that; to do this, and to stop doing that! All the things that we are doing wrong, eating wrong, understanding wrong, and all that we need to do right!

Fad diets are everywhere! Some tell us to eat in moderations, others to eat almost nothing at all; some lead us to the path of health, others only guide us to lose weight and look thin. It is very easy to get confused about exactly which one diet could be the right one for us.

The Mediterranean Diet may be new in the diet industry, but it has been in circulation for thousands of years. As the name suggests, this diet follows the dietary habit of the countries around the Mediterranean Sea, particularly of Italy and France, but mainly of Greece. Eat as the ancient Greeks used to eat, apparently!

This diet could be considered quite different from a number of other diets that are popular these days, mainly because the limitations are not so strict here. Neither the amount of food to be eaten nor the types of food that can be eaten is limited much here. Unlike most other diets out there, the Mediterranean diet is fast gaining popularity because of the freedom it allows its followers.

Yes, this is definitely a diet that deserves our attention!

So, read on if you want to learn more about the Mediterranean Diet, because everything that you need to know about this diet can be found in this book. Good luck on your quest!

Chapter 1: Know the Mediterranean Diet

The ancient Greeks had given us Homer, the Iliad and the Odyssey, mythology; they have paved the way for democracy and fashion, the Olympics and theater.

The Romans have given us architecture, Latin, the calendar, books and highways. The French had always led the way in fashion, art, philosophy and literature.

Yes, these 3, and the other 11 countries with borders in the Mediterranean Sea have always been pioneers in so many ways, but did we ever think that one day we'll also be following their dietary habits? Why not? We've always loved the rich and aromatic Mediterranean cuisine! What could be better than to add these dishes to our regular diet so that we can be healthier and happier?

What is the Mediterranean Diet?

Basically, the Mediterranean Diet is to follow the dietary habits of the inhabitants of the Mediterranean countries in the

1940s, 1950s and 1960s, before fast food made an appearance in these countries.

Diets in these countries, from the ancient times, have been diverse and delicious. There is no "one diet" that all these countries practice, but a general pattern that they follow. The Greek cuisine is completely different from the Egyptian cuisine, as is French food different from Spanish dishes; but there are, or there was before the 1970s, certain guidelines that these countries follow.

It is not the particular cuisine that is important in this diet, but some of the main ingredients that most of these countries include in their regular meals that sets them apart from every other diet, and that's what we need to learn more about.

Why the Mediterranean Diet?

Now, that is a good question! Why the Mediterranean diet, when there are so many others that support the modern Western lifestyle? This is because statistics show that the inhabitants of these countries - particularly Greece, France and Italy - have better health than most countries of the west.

Multiple studies have shown that people who follow the Mediterranean Diet - who actually adopt this diet completely in their lives without fail - have been known to have lower risks of developing a number of diseases and health problems.

Most of the modern population living in cities work hard in office jobs, stay in front of the computer all day long, eat processed and packaged foods, and exercise as less as possible. Most of them are also worried about obesity and heart diseases, Type-II diabetes and cholesterol. Mediterranean diet, on the other hand, emphasizes hard on staying active and eating fresh and home-cooked food.

According to the Center for Disease Control and Prevention, over 610,000 people die of heart diseases every year in the United States of America. This comes down to 1 in every 4 people who have died from different kind of cardio vascular diseases, more in men than women. At the same time, more than 735,000 people in the USA suffer from heart attacks in America annually, an astounding number.

In 1958, Professor Ancel Keys, a physiologist from Minnesota, conducted The Seven Countries Study, in which he came to the conclusion that both the rates of death and heart diseases in some of the Mediterranean countries - particularly Greece, Crete and Italy - were significantly lower than the rates in USA, UK and Finland. After further investigation into the lifestyles of the people of these countries, he accomplished that it was mainly because of their dietary habits that they are healthier and fitter nations.

Other studies has shown that eating a daily meal full of fruits and vegetables, as is possible by following the Mediterranean Diet, it is possible to lower the levels of low-density lipoprotein, or LDL, in your blood. LDL is known as the "bad" cholesterol, lowering which leads to lower deposits inside your arteries.

Besides, inhabitants of the Mediterranean countries have been known to have longer lives, mainly .because they have a significantly lower chance of any heart diseases or heart attacks. Not only that, this diet can also work wonders in battling depression, obesity, Alzheimer's Disease, dementia, a number of types of cancer, Type-II diabetes and Parkinson's Disease. For women, incorporating Mediterranean Diet into their lives can significantly reduce the chances of breast cancer.

In a study conducted by at the Department of Nutrition, Harvard School of Public Health, the main investigator, Dr. Walter Willet, concluded that, "Together with regular physical activity and no smoking, our analysis suggests that over 80% of coronary heart disease, 70% of strokes and 90% of Type-II diabetes can be avoided by healthy food choices that are consistent with the traditional Mediterranean diet."

Because of the inactive life we lead, it is very easy to contact a number of diseases, especially Type-II diabetes and obesity. What's unique about the Mediterranean diet is that it doesn't only give us an idea about what to eat, but puts a huge emphasis on leading an active life.

Mainly because of this dual combination of healthy eating and living an active life, the Mediterranean diet is considered as one of the healthiest lifestyle choices out there!

History of the Mediterranean Diet

Like the cuisine, the history of the Mediterranean diet is also colorful and full of flavors!

The Mediterranean basin, where the borders of more than 20 countries lie, was called "the cradle of society" by historians, mainly because this is where most of the important ancient civilizations started. The Egyptian, Sumerian, Assyrian, Babylonian and Persian civilizations all started along this basin, although any information about their dietary habits has been long lost in time.

From old Greek scriptures, we find an idea of their daily meals - bread, cheese, fruits and vegetables for the middle class while the rich and powerful favored seafood, fresh fish, red meat and good wine. The slaves had to be happy with dry bread and olives, and a little salted fish if they were lucky. Hardly nutritious, but that was their daily diet for hundreds of years! The Roman culture soon blended with the Greek lifestyle and opened up new opportunities in hunting, gathering and farming. Households began raising pigs for fat and growing vegetables and a little amount of grain in their kitchen gardens. Red meat cooked in fat entered every family along with home grown vegetables and beer made from grains.

It was the Muslims that brought in the culture of extended agriculture to the Mediterranean basin, but they could only be afforded by the wealthy and the influential. The introduction of sugarcane, eggplant, oranges, lemon, almonds, citrus, rice and spinach led to new recipes and variety of tastes.

When the Europeans discovered America, they also discovered tomatoes, potatoes, corn and chili - ingredients that were widely popular there. The tomato, which later became a significant part of Mediterranean cuisine, was a surprisingly late introduction to this area.

Although Mediterranean diet can seen a number of changes all throughout history - from the time of the ancient civilizations to the later invasion of new lands - its ideology and basic has always been the same. Where the rest of the whole is slowly growing dependent on packaged and processed food, the countries along the Mediterranean basin has always believed in the wholesomeness of home-cooked and personally-prepared food.

This is particularly why the Mediterranean diet is becoming widely popular around the world, because deep within, everyone loves to sit down to lovingly prepared food that is good for them and their family members.

Chapter 2: The Basics of a Mediterranean Diet

The modern world has a number of misconceptions about Mediterranean food. To us, they represent cheese pizza, oven-baked pasta, cheese and bread, wine, and the Caesar Salad. We all love what they have to offer to a generation who loves to live on carb and proteins!

In truth, all that we know about Greek, French and Italian cuisine, as well as about the other countries around this part of the world, is only a part of what Mediterranean cuisine is. To eat as in Mediterranean countries is not to dine on pizza and pasta, or to eat cheese and bread for breakfast, lunch and dinner!

Understanding the Mediterranean Diet

The basics of Mediterranean Diet are simple and easy - eat fresh, eat healthy, eat well! When something is good for you, eat them every day and as much as you can. Don't entirely leave out what might not be too good for you, but consume them in moderation. Be active, be merry, and eat with your family and friends around you!

With the Mediterranean diet, you don't just consume food. You prepare, cook, serve, eat food with your loved ones. Eating as well as cooking is supposed to something to enjoy and look forward to, not just something you have to do because you need to live!

This diet focuses as much as on enjoying food as it does on health and wellbeing. This is probably why people everywhere love the Mediterranean diet, because we all love food, that's for sure!

To understand how the Mediterranean diet works, you have to first understand its basic ideology and rules. The first thing that you need to know about the Mediterranean diet is that your main focus should be on plants. Besides the obvious fruits and vegetables, a plant-based diet also includes whole grains, nuts and legumes, seeds and beans.

Fish and other seafood come in after plants, but only in moderation, and not every day. The place for poultry and dairy comes after that, and finally there is provision for meat and sweets.

So you see, a Mediterranean diet is not just about a large pepperoni pizza and pita and hummus. There's a lot that this diet has to offer that is good for your health, but also gives you the freedom to plan your meals to your liking.

The Mediterranean Diet Pyramid

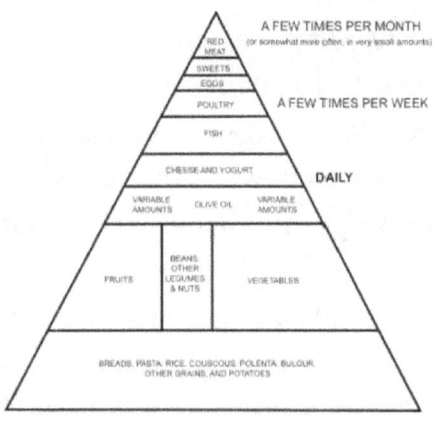

This diet follows a specific pyramid-shaped model that makes it easier for you to understand the basics. It describes all the types of food allowed under the Mediterranean diet, and in what frequency.

As you can see from the pyramid above, our present diet is quite the opposite. We prefer steaks to fruits every day, and order desserts with every meal. We eat eggs for breakfast instead of grains, and we snack on packaged and fast foods. No wonder more than half the population of the world is unhealthy and unfit!

To follow the Mediterranean diet, your daily meals need to be a balanced combination of grain-based food, i.e. bread, pasta and rice, as well as adequate amounts of fruits, vegetables and nuts. Fish, seafood and dairy should be in your menu only few times a week; lean meat and sweets should be limited to as little as a few times in a month.

This is how people living in the Mediterranean countries have been eating for hundreds of year. They prefer home-cooked meals to the ones that need to be micro-waved, and they include fresh fruits and vegetables in their daily meals rather than deep-fried and oily food. This pyramid is the reason that people living in the Mediterranean basin has been healthy and happy for so many generations.

Basic Elements of the Mediterranean Diet

To make the diet simpler and more interesting, there are a few basic information that you need to understand and keep in mind.

- It's a plant-based diet

The Mediterranean diet is, first and foremost, a plant-based diet. Most of the food that the inhabitants of Mediterranean countries eat regularly comes from plants - directly or altered. Fruits are consumed raw and vegetables are cooked and made into salads. At the same time, seeds and nuts are widely popular as snacks or in cooked dishes.

- Carbohydrates are allowed

Most diets strictly leave out all forms of carbohydrates, but not all carb are bad for you. There are some healthy carbohydrates that are included in everyday meals with the Mediterranean diet, i.e. whole-grains and beans. These healthy carbohydrates, when introduced to your diet moderately, would not add to your weight, but keep you healthy.

- Only healthy fats are used

Just like carb, not all fats are unhealthy. Oil extracted from olives is considered to be one of the healthiest forms of fats available in nature. Olive oil is essential for all types of Mediterranean cuisine, from pizza to salad. This oil helps in lowering cholesterol and can be used liberally in cooking.

Unhealthy sources of fat such as butter, margarine or cooking oil, on the other hand, actually increases cholesterol level in blood and damage the arteries, no matter how little is used.

- Herbs and spices are important

Instead of adding sugar and salt to bring flavor, Mediterranean cuisines use natural herbs and spices, like garlic and ginger, basil, citrus juice, sugarcane juice, cinnamon, sage, pepper, etc. Almost all of these herbs and spices have a number of good effects on our body that cannot be achieved with refined sugar or salt.

- Animal Protein is consumed moderately

Lean protein and fish should be only eaten once or twice a week, and in moderation. In forms of KFC or meatloaf, pizza or steak - meat has become a part of our everyday life in this modern world, which is unimaginable in the Mediterranean countries. Seafood, fishes and meat dishes can be seen on the table only twice or at most, three times a week.

Fish is the main source of animal protein in Mediterranean households, not chicken or beef. A small serving of fish can be allowed up to three times a week; chicken and other animal protein less than that. Red meat is almost absent from Mediterranean recipes, and may only be consumed on special occasions, and less than 3 ounces.

- Dairy and poultry are limited, too

Dairy and poultry, i.e. cheese, milk, butter, margarine and eggs - are a daily part of our lives. In the Mediterranean diet, however, dairy and poultry is limited to only three to four times a week, that too, in small potions.

- Healthy desserts are served

In Mediterranean households, most desserts are inspired by fruits, and made from fruit. Sugar or artificial sweetener is almost never used; fruit dishes are sweetened with natural herbs and spices. Desserts high in sweeteners are allowed once or twice a month, but only in small portions and mostly on special occasions.

- It's okay to drink what's allowed

Water should be your main drink with the Mediterranean diet - pure, room temperature, unsweetened water. Citrus water and fruit juices are also common, but only when you don't add any sugar or sweetener to it.

Beside water, a little consumption of red wine every day is considered to be healthy in the Mediterranean countries. 1 serving of drink (around 0.5 cup) for women and 2 servings for men is recommended and practiced. Drinks should not be taken on an empty stomach, especially if you have diabetes, low blood glucose or hypoglycemia.

Apart from the restrictions of what can be eaten and what should be avoided, there are some other elements of the Mediterranean diet that are unique.

- It's important to be physically active

One of the most important elements of the Mediterranean diet is its emphasis on living an active life.

The Mediterranean diet is basically a reflection of the "poor man's diet" living in this region for thousands of years, and if anything, they were hardworking. The common people living in the Mediterranean basin worked hard for their living - manual labor, not the office work we are used to now. In order to make this diet successful, we need to be active. Although manual labor may not be possible for everyone, it is certainly possible to walk, jog and run, exercise and dance regularly.

Being physically active is a significant part of the Mediterranean lifestyle, and to make this diet a success, we need to involve in more and more physical activities.

- It's important to limit your portions

The Mediterranean diet pyramid comes into focus here. The food items from the bottom of the pyramid can be consumed in larger portions - fruits and vegetables, whereas the portions slowly start decreasing as you climb to the upper layers of the pyramid, towards meat and dessert. It's not only portion sizes that you need to control when you reach the upper levels of the pyramid, but also how many times you serve them during the week or month.

To maintain your portions and servings is an important element of the Mediterranean diet, one that is integral in your success with this diet.

- It's important to eat in moderation

The Mediterranean diet doesn't ask you to completely let go of everything that you love but is unhealthy; it's just that you need to limit your consumptions to a moderate amount. Birthday cakes are fine twice a month, but only if you take a small slice; enjoying a steak with your family and friends is completely fine on the odd weekends, but not if you start having steak regularly.

- It's important to cook and eat with others

People living in the Mediterranean countries understand the importance of cooking and eating with friends and family, instead of by themselves in front of the television. For them, the entire act of preparing, cooking, serving and eating - even cleaning up - should be done with others present, amid laughter and conversations.

Cooking and eating in Mediterranean households are a family affair. Simple and easy dishes are prepared with friends and every meal is enjoyed in the company of others. Physical activities are encouraged, even if it is in the form of simply walking or dancing. Fresh and home-cooked meals are most preferred, as are fruits and vegetables. These unique elements of the Mediterranean diet are what's making this diet a favorite among health conscious population of the world.

Chapter 3: Planning a Mediterranean Diet

If you are new to the concept of a Mediterranean diet, it would be difficult for you to actually start the diet based on the rules and regulations alone. What you need is an in-depth discussion about this diet - a complete list of what you can and cannot eat, what's allowed and what's not, as well as an absolute idea of what your kitchen, refrigerator and pantry should look like.

All of which you will find ready in this chapter.

What to Eat

Let us assure you that you will find a lot to eat under the Mediterranean diet. You won't have to go through the torture of sticking to 2/3 ingredients every day and avoid everything else. Yes, if your daily diet consisted on a doughnut for breakfast, steak for lunch and pizza for dinner - you might have to make quite some changes. But if you were already living a relatively healthy life with lots of greens, the transition to better health will be easy for you.

Here is a complete list of everything that you can eat when you are following the Mediterranean diet.

Fruits

Apples, pears, oranges, banana, dates, grapes, avocado, figs, peaches, melons, apricots, clementines, strawberries, plums, pomegranates, pineapples, tangerines, cherries, and of course, olives are regularly eaten in the Mediterranean countries. However, remember that some fruits - like banana and cherries - are sweet and high in sugar and should be limited a little more than other fruits that are mostly fiber and water, like watermelon and figs.

There's nothing better than fresh and whole fruits - especially seasonal ones that are readily available in the Mediterranean countries all through the year. Fruit juices are great for quenching your thirst on a hot summer day, but they lack the fiber of the actual fruit the juice is extracted from. So, if possible, you should try to consume the whole fruit rather than fruit juices, but only when they are natural, fresh and completely unsweetened.

Vegetables

Broccoli, spinach, kale, all kinds of onions - red, white and sweet, cauliflowers and cabbages, carrots, Brussels' sprouts, arugula, carrots and cucumbers, courgettes, leeks, asparagus, peppers, lettuce, artichokes, mache, radishes, scallions, peas, potatoes, chicory, eggplant, collard greens, dandelions and fennel, lemons and of course tomatoes are grown in kitchen gardens all over the Mediterranean countries and used regularly in meals.

Most vegetables are cooked with olive oil, while some are used in crunchy summer salads for lunch and dinner. Vegetables in these countries are not only a side dish to be served with meat or steak, but the staple food that are seen on the table every day, all through the year.

Grains

Not all sources of carbohydrate are bad and make you gain weight; rather whole grains are good for your metabolism. A limited but regular intake of whole grains can lower your "bad" blood, regulate your bowel movements, and decrease chances of cancer.

Wheat, rye, barley and brown rice, oats and corn in a small amount every day can be a good thing for you. Grains in form of spaghetti, cereals, corn flakes, whole meal pasta and bread, porridge, biscuits, polenta, couscous and muesli can become a part of your regular meals, but in very limited amount.

Beans and Legumes

Other important ingredients in Mediterranean cuisine are beans and legumes; all kinds of beans - fava, kidney, cannellini and green, as well as chickpeas, lentils, tahini and pulses are regularly used in their dishes. These beans and legumes are used in cooking as well as salad, and helps in adding texture and color to their dishes.

Nuts and Seeds

Nuts and seeds are used mostly as snacks, or in salads to add an extra crunch to them. All kinds of nuts - cashew nut, peanut, almonds, hazelnuts, pistachio and pine nuts, and walnuts are favorite snack of the Mediterranean countries to chew in leisure moments, as are sunflower and sesame seeds.

Herbs and Spices

Traditional herbs and spices are used in Mediterranean cuisine mainly to reduce the need for adding extra fat, salt or sugar. Sea salt is used as an alternative to refined salt; cinnamon and sugarcane extract instead of sugar. Other common and popular herbs and spices include sage, turmeric, cumin, fennel, cloves, lavender, garlic and ginger, rosemary, bay leaf, chili and pepper, lavender, mint, marjoram, parsley, oregano, thyme, za'atar and sumac, terragon and savory.

Some of the above mentioned herbs and spices are common and known to us; but it is the uncommon condiments that add the unique Mediterranean flavor to their vegetable dishes, salads and savory desserts.

After the staple fruits, vegetables, grains and other such ingredients, come the lesser important sources of protein, dairy and poultry.

Fish and Seafood

Fish and Seafood are the main sources of animal protein in the Mediterranean diet, not meat. Almost all kinds of fishes are regularly consumed by the people living in these regions, mostly salmons and sardines, tuna, mackerel, tilapia, yellowtail, trout, flounders and eels. Among seafood, clams, crabs and cockles, lobsters, octopuses, oysters, sea bass, shrimps and whelk are popular and widely loved.

Seafood and fish dishes are prepared twice or thrice a week in Mediterranean households, and enjoyed by everyone. Fried, cooked, steamed or used in salads - they are healthy and delicious at all times! Most of the fishes consumed in these countries are rich in Omega-3 fatty acids, which is good for the heart.

Poultry and Dairy

Most of the poultry and dairy items that we consume every day go unnoticed by us - the cheese in a pizza, a portion of egg in our morning sandwich, the milk with a whole-grain cereal. In reality, we are eating poultry and dairy one way or other every day!

In traditional Mediterranean households, milk, cheese, eggs and yogurt is consumed not more than twice or thrice a week. The calcium found in dairy and poultry goods are great for bones, heart and your overall health in forms of feta cheese, corvo, ricotta, Greek and regular yogurt, brie, manchego, parmesan, pecorino and haloumi.

Eggs from chicken, quall and ducks - all are common in Mediterranean households.

Meat

Meat in lean cut and minimum proportions are served not more than three or four times per month, which comes down to once a week. Chicken, duck and guinea fowl are more common than beef, pork, lamb, mutton or goat.

Cuts are important in determining the food value of meat protein. People of this region prefer their meat to be lean cut with as less saturated fat as possible. When ground meat is used in recipes, it is usually 90% lean meat and 10% fat - which is as healthy as it is delicious to cook with.

Drinks

Your most preferred form of drink should be water, as mentioned earlier in this book. Water at room temperature is better than chilled water for your health, but sometimes, cold water on a hot day is fine.

Water keeps your body hydrated, and in countries of the Mediterranean region, it is very important to drink plenty of water so keep healthy. Especially when a person leads an active life under the harsh sun, plenty of water becomes an important part of their daily diet. The standard amount of water necessary for an able-bodied adult would be 8-10 glasses a day, but more depending on the person's size, weight and physical activities.

Wine, particularly red wine, in moderation is also common among families living in the Mediterranean region, except in countries where drinking is frowned upon because of religious reasons. Other types of alcoholic beverages are also available in these countries, but it's the different types of wines that are more loved by locals.

Fats

Only olive oil and avocado oil are used in Mediterranean cuisine, in cooking, salads, snacks and even in desserts. Extra virgin olive oil is considered to be the healthiest fat there is and preferred by most Mediterranean families in preparing their food.

What Not to Eat

If you can just keep in mind that fresh and home-cooked meals are better for your health, you won't have to worry much about making the transition to a Mediterranean lifestyle.

Added Sugars

Food items that are rich in added sugar and sweeteners, mainly processed foods like soda, chocolate bars, candy, ice cream, cookies, etc should be completely avoided.

Trans Fat

Trans fat is found in margarine, frozen pizzas, pie crusts and cakes, and is extremely bad for your health.

Processed Meat

A little amount of meat is fine, but not when they are processed and packaged in the form of sausages and hot dog meat.

Refined Grains

White bread, white rice, white or all-purpose flour, white pasta - these are all refined grains and can add to your weight.

Refined Oil

Any other type of oil other than olive and avocado oil, i.e. soybean oil, canola oil, cottonseed and other vegetable oil is refined and should be avoided.

In short, almost everything that comes in packages, made in factories or contain the words "low-fat" and "diet" should be avoided as much as possible, if not completely.

Chapter 4: 7-Day Mediterranean Meal Plan

Now that you have an idea of the kind of ingredients you need to bring home or yourself and your family, what you need is a week-long meal plan that you can adopt to try out a Mediterranean lifestyle.

Mediterranean meal plans would ideally be varied, since there are so many recipes to choose from. A few servings of dairy and poultry each week, and mostly fruits, vegetables and whole grains for breakfast, lunch and dinner, seafood and fish not more than a few times in a week, and rarely any meat or desserts - that's what an ideal Mediterranean diet should consist.

Day-1

Let's call this week the "Day of Zeus", after the Greek God from where Greek mythology starts. Zeus was the father of most of the prominent Gods and Goddesses of Greek mythology, and his story is where all myths of this era start. We start our Mediterranean diet with this day, just like we start Greek Mythology with learning about Zeus.

- For breakfast, let's start our Mediterranean lifestyle with something we all love - fluffy and soft pancakes made from some old-fashioned oats.
- For lunch, a Greek-styled salad completely light but filling salad that you can prepare and eat anywhere, and absolutely love.
- For dinner, eat like the king that Zeus was, with chicken thighs stuffed with tomato sauce.

- If you are hungry in the evenings, a snack of herbed olives will keep you happy.

Day-2

We'll call this day the "Day of Poseidon" because the special dish of the day is a seafood dish dedicated to the God of the Seas - Poseidon.

- For breakfast, a light start of the day with crunchy toast with an avocado spread.

For lunch, a chicken salad with herbs, cooked in Greek style, to celebrate our favorite powerful Gods of Greek mythology.

Finally for dinner, to celebrate the "Day of Poseidon", a touch of fish, cooked Mediterranean style, that will liven up your dinner plans. Perfect for the whole family or if you have friends over; everyone will love this Mediterranean-styled fish fillet.

For the little hungers in the middle of the day, as many roasted chickpeas as you can eat as a snack.

Day-3
Let's call the third day "The Day of Hestia" after the Greek Goddess of domesticity, the hearth, the family and the household. On the day of Hestia, we will be eating homely food with ingredients that can be found inside the house.
- For breakfast, a filling omelet - healthy and nutritious, made with cheese and vegetables!
- For lunch, pasta salad made from whole-grain pasta, cheese and lots of your favorite vegetables.
- For dinner, whole grilled tomatoes stuffed with croutons and cheese.
- For your midnight snacking needs, fresh blueberries covered with cream.

Day-4

We'll call the 4th day "The Day of Ares" after the Greek God of war, because we'll be start the day as if preparing for war!

For breakfast, a heavy breakfast of couscous - perfect for a fulfilling meal to get you ready for the long day ahead.
For lunch, panzanella - a healthy meal of whole-grain bread, tomatoes and cheese.

For dinner, a heavy meal of chicken thighs stuffed with tomato sauce to give you some much-needed animal protein.
As a snack for a trying day, some pears poached in fruit juice - a healthy dessert!

Day-5

We'll call the 4th day "The Day of Athena" after the Greek Goddess of wisdom, intelligence, strategic planning and intellectual beauty, because you need some wholesome food to go through the day.

For breakfast, a heavy breakfast of banana-and-nut oatmeal, a breakfast that will help you think and plan clearly.

For lunch, soup of white bean that will give you further mental strength and stability for the day.

Chickpea patties for dinner, something fried and filling made from nutritious legumes and vegetables.

A snack of delicious tomato skewers with cheese balls and basil when you are hungry.

Day-6
We'll call the 6th day the "Day of Demeter" - after this beautiful and bountiful Goddess of agriculture and harvest, because we are going to spend this day as a vegetarian.
- For breakfast, a frittata with zucchini and goat cheese - a vegetarian breakfast that is filling and delicious.
- For lunch, grilled vegetable tagine made from potatoes and tomatoes.

- For dinner, a delicious meal of stuffed tomatoes.
- If you are looking for a snack, there's an option of olives marinated in herbs and served with feta cheese.

Day-7

Day 7 is the "Day of Hera" - the Greek Goddess of motherhood, marriage and families. This is the day that you are going to cook for and with your whole family, and enjoy wholesome food that everyone will love and look forward to eating.

- For breakfast, a parfait made from berries and yogurt!

- For lunch, a sandwich, but one that has eggplants in it. Strange? Just try it once and you'll never go back to a normal sandwich again!
- For dinner, amazingly, pizza!

- For a snack or a dessert after dinner, yummy rice pudding.

If these names sound delicious to you, check out the next chapter where you will find easy and quick recipes for each of them that you can make at home without any trouble.

Chapter 5: Mediterranean Diet Recipes

Mediterranean recipes are quick, easy, simple and fresh. In short, the cuisines from the countries around the Mediterranean basin are not just healthy, they are wholesome. Every cuisine from these countries reflects their culture, their wealth and family life, as well as their tradition.

In these chapter are some of the most beloved recipes of this region according to the 7-day meal for you and your family from the previous chapter.

For Breakfast

Breakfast has always been the most important meal of the day, even when you are on a diet. With the Mediterranean diet, you can have a wide choice of breakfast meals - from classic pancakes and omelets, to more exotic dishes like couscous and frittatas.

Soft and Fluffy Pancakes

Ingredients:

- 2 cups of whole oats
- 1 cup of whole-grain wheat flour
- 2 tablespoons of baking soda
- 4 tablespoons of flax seeds
- 4 large eggs
- 4 cups of yogurt, plain
- 4 tablespoon of honey
- 4 tablespoon of olive oil
- Fresh fruit, as toppings

Directions:

- Combine the oats, flour, baking soda, flax seeds and salt in a blender.
- Blend together till everything becomes dust-like together.
- Add the eggs, yogurt, honey and oil to it.

- Blend together for another minute or more.
- Let the batter thicken by keeping it standing for 25-30 minutes.
- Heat a large pan.
- Brush some olive oil into the pan.
- Each time, pour 1/4th cup of batter on the heated pan in perfect circles.
- Wait until the bottom part of the pancake is brown and hard.
- Turn the pancake over using a spoon.
- Cook on medium heat until both sides resemble each other.
- Serve hot with your favorite fruits as toppings.

Servings: 10

Avocado with Toast

Who says you can't have toast just because you are on a healthy diet? With this recipe, you can have your share of yummy toast for breakfast.

Ingredients:

- 8 slices of whole-grain rye bread
- 4 small avocados, peeled and pitted

- 1/2 cups of feta cheese, crumbled
- 4 tablespoons of fresh mint, finely chopped
- 4 teaspoon of lemon juice, freshly squeezed
- Sea salt and pepper, to taste.
- 8 slices of ham (Optional)

Direction:
- In a bowl, mash the avocado with a fork.
- Add the chopped mint and lemon juice.
- Mix together.
- Season with your preferred amount of salt and pepper.
- Grill or toast the rye bread to your preferred crispiness.
- Spoon out 1/8th of the avocado spread on to individual pieces of toast.
  - Sprinkle the crumbled feta cheese on top.

Servings: 4

Greek-styled Omelet

Start your day with a filling omelet that will keep you full till the late hours for lunch.

Ingredients:

- 8 large eggs
- 1/2 cup of spinach, cooked in water
- 1 cup of feta cheese, crumbled
- 4 teaspoons of dill, freshly chopped
- 2 tablespoon of olive oil, extra-virgin
- 4 scallions, sliced
- Pepper to taste, freshly ground

Directions:

- In a bowl, mix the eggs together well.
- Add the crumbled feta cheese, dill, scallions and pepper.
- Mix well.
- Squeeze the spinach to remove any excess water, and add to the eggs.
- Preheat a skillet and brush with olive oil.
- Pour in the egg mixture, half at a time.
- Tilt the skillet to distribute the eggs evenly.

- Cook the eggs until the bottom is hard and golden brown.
- Turn over the egg and cook until both sides look the same.
  - Cook for 2 to 3 minutes and serve on individual plates.

Servings: 4

Breakfast Couscous

When you have a long and important day ahead of you, you need a heavy breakfast to start the day. A fulfilling meal of couscous - a popular Moroccan dish, will do just that for you!

Ingredients:

- 2 cups of whole-grain couscous, uncooked
- 5 cups of milk, low-fat or fat-free
- 1 cup of apricots, dried
- 1/2 cup of currants, dried
- 4 tablespoons of butter, melted
  (Note: if you are not comfortable with butter, substitute with olive oil)
- 10 tablespoons of honey

- 2 cinnamon sticks, 1/2 inch each
- 1/2 teaspoon of sea salt

Direction:

- Heat the milk in a large pan over low fire.
- Add the cinnamon sticks and cook for 5 minutes.

  (Note: Do not let the milk come to a boil.)
- Remove the milk from over the fire.
- Add the uncooked couscous, honey, salt, apricots and currents.
  - Cover and pan and let stand for 20 minutes.
  - Find and discard the cinnamon sticks.
  - Serve equally in four individual bowls.

Servings: 4

Banana-and-Nut Oatmeal

A classic breakfast of oatmeal, fruit and nuts to have a great start of the day!

Ingredients:

- 1/2 cup of cooking oat
- 1 cup milk, skim or fat-free
- 1 medium sized banana, peeled
- 4 tablespoons of walnuts, chopped
- 1 teaspoon of flax seeds
- 6 tablespoons of honey

Direction:
- In a bowl safe for the microwave, combine the milk, oats and honey.
- Add the walnuts and the flax seeds.
- Cook in the microwave on high heat for 3 minutes.
- Use a fork to thoroughly mash the banana.
- Add the mashed banana to the oatmeal.
- Serve warm from the microwave oven.

Servings: 2

Zucchini Frittata with Goat Cheese
A spicy and delicious breakfast recipe for the whole family to enjoy on a relaxed weekend at home!
Ingredients:
- 8 large eggs, *whisked*
- 4 tablespoons of milk, *fat free*

- 2 medium-sized zucchini
- 3 ounces of goat cheese, *crumbled*
- 1 clove of garlic, *minced*
- 2 tablespoons of olive oil, *extra virgin*
- 1/2 teaspoon of sea salt
- 1/4 teaspoon of pepper

Direction:
- Preheat the oven to 350°F.
- Slice the zucchini into round slices, each 1/4 inch in height.
- In the bowl, combine the milk with salt and pepper.
- Whisk well to mix.
- In a skillet that is ovenproof, heat olive oil.
- Add the garlic and cook for 1 minute.
- Add the zucchini slices and cook for another 5 minutes.
- Pour the whisked egg into the skillet.
- Stir cook for 2 minutes.
- Add the goat cheese to the pan and stir.
- Transfer the skillet to the oven, and bake for 15 minutes until the egg is set.
- Remove and let sit for 5 minutes outside.

- Slice frittata into 4 slices and serve in individual plates.

Servings: 4

Berries-and-Yogurt Parfait

A light breakfast that you can enjoy with your whole family that everyone will love!
Ingredients:
- 4 cups of yogurt, low fat or fat free
- 1 cup of fresh strawberries, with juice
- 1 cup of fresh blueberries (or blackberries or raspberries), with juice
- 2 cups of granola, whole-wheat
- Direction:
- Take 4 individual tall glasses wide enough to insert spoons.
- Pour in 1/2 cup of vanilla yogurt into each glass.
- Add a combination of berries into the glasses.
- Add 1/2 cup of granola over the berries.
- Pour in another 1/2 cup of yogurt on top of the granola.

- Top off with an assortment of berries until the glasses are full.
- Serve immediately so that the granola remains crunchy.

Servings: 4

Lunch

Lunches are usually light and quick meals in the middle of a busy day, either at work or at home. Hardworking people prefer their lunches to be either a light salad or a sandwich, or something equally simple.

Greek-styled Salad

Ingredients:
- 1 Romanian lettuce, head only
- 1 cup of feta cheese, crumbled
- 1 bell pepper (green), chopped
- 1 bell pepper (red), chopped
- 1 cucumber, sliced
- 2 tomatoes (large), chopped
- 1 red onion, chopped
- 6 ounces of olives, pitted
- 1 lemon, freshly squeezed
- 1 teaspoon of oregano, dried

- 6 tablespoons of olive oil,
- Black Pepper to taste, ground

Directions:

- Combine all the vegetables together in a large salad bowl.
- In a separate bowl, combine the oregano, olive oil, black pepper and lemon juice.
- Whisk together to mix.
- Pour the dressing mixture over the vegetables.
- Toss together to mix and serve fresh.

Serving: 8

Greek Chicken Salad with Herbs

After a whole day of abstaining, you must be craving for some animal-based protein! Here's a light chicken salad to realize that craving and fill you up.

Ingredients:

- 2 pound of chicken (boneless), cut into small cubes
- 2 cups of yogurt (plain)
- 4 teaspoons of tahini

- 12 cups of Romanian lettuce, chopped
- 2 cups of English cucumber, chopped
- 2 cups of tomatoes, halved
- 1/2 cup of feta cheese, crumbled
- 10 olives, pitted
- 2 teaspoons of garlic, minced
- 1 teaspoon of garlic powder
- 2 teaspoon of oregano, dried
- 2 teaspoons of black pepper, ground
- 1 teaspoon of sea salt
- 2 teaspoons of olive oil

Directions:

- Mix the oregano, garlic powder, and half the pepper and salt in a bowl.
- Heat a medium sized pan.
- Pour in the olive oil and tilt to distribute evenly.
- Add the chicken.
- Add the mixed spices to the chicken.
- Sauté over medium heat until the chicken is cooked.
- Add half the lemon juice and remove from the fire.

- Mix together the rest of lemon juice with the remaining salt and pepper, tahini, yogurt and garlic.
- Stir together to mix well.
- In a large salad bowl, combine all the chopped vegetables together.
- Serve 2 cups of salad to individual plates.
- Add 1/2 cup of cooked chicken to each plate.
- Mix well and drizzle the spiced yogurt mixture on each plate.

Servings: 6

Pasta Salad

Finally, a dish that resembles our idea of Italian cuisine, but one that is also healthy!
Ingredients:

- 10 ounces of whole-grain pasta, any kind you like
- 10 ounces of skim mozzarella cheese, chopped
- 15 ounces of artichoke hearts (from a can), drained and dried
- 1/2 cup of red bell pepper, chopped

- 1/2 cup of peas, frozen
- 1/2 cup of parsley, chopped
- 1 lemon, freshly squeezed
- 4 tablespoons of olive oil

Direction:

- Cook the pasta in water, but without any salt or oil.
- Mix the lemon juice and olive oil together in a separate large bowl.
- Add the artichoke hearts, bell peppers, cheese and parsley to the bowl.
- Toss for a few minutes to mix well.
- Drain the cooked pasta and the peas together in a colander.
- (Note: Don't run under cold water.)
- Add the pasta and the peas to the salad.
- Toss to mix well.
- Serve warm or cold depending on your preference.

Servings: 4

Panzanella

A delicious Sicilian recipe that everybody loves, and that will bring an abundance of colors and flavors to your table.

Ingredients:

- 2 cups of whole-wheat bread, toasted and cubed
- 2 cups of tomatoes, chopped
- 1 cup of cucumber, chopped
- 1/2 cup of red onions, chopped
- 1/4 cup of feta cheese, crumbled
- 2 tablespoons of red wine
- 2 teaspoons of olive oil, extra virgin
- 1 teaspoon of black pepper, ground

Direction:

- Cut the toasts into small cubes, each of 1 inch.
- Add the tomatoes, cucumbers, red onion and feta cheese.
- Toss together to mix well.
- Sprinkle the vinegar, olive oil and pepper to the salad.
- Keep covered in a bowl in room temperature for 3-4 hours.

- Serve at room temperature without heating.

    Servings: 2

White Bean Soup

An Italian delicacy that is healthy, and that will give you the energy to face the day!
Ingredients:
- 16 ounces of white kidney beans (from a can), rinsed and dried
- 14 ounces of broth, vegetable or chicken
- 1 bunch of spinach, thinly sliced
- 1 red onion, chopped
- 1 clove of garlic, chopped
- 1 stalk of celery, chopped
- 1/2 teaspoon of black pepper, ground
- A pinch of thyme, dried
- 1 tablespoon of lemon juice, freshly squeezed
- 2 tablespoon of olive oil, extra virgin
- 2 cups of water

Direction:
- Heat oil in a large pot over medium fire.

- Cook the onions and the celery in hot oil until tender.
- Add the minced garlic and cook for another 2 minutes.
- Add the white beans, broth, thyme, pepper and water to the pot.
- Bring to a boil.
- Reduce the heat and let the soup simmer for 20 minutes.
- Remove 2 cups of beans and vegetables from the soup and set aside.
- Add the rest of the soup to a blender.
- Blend until smooth.
- Return the blended soup to the pot and cook in low heat.
- Add the beans and vegetables previously set aside.
- Bring the soup to a slow boil over low heat.
- Add the sliced spinach leaves.
- Cook for another 3 minutes.
- Add the lemon juice to the pot.
- Remove the pot from heat.
- Let stand for 2 minutes before serving.
- Serve hot.

(Note: You can grate some parmesan cheese on top before serving)

Servings: 4

Grilled Vegetable Tagine

An all-vegetable recipe, very light and appetizing - when you have a long day ahead to focus on.

Ingredients:
- 30 ounces of tomatoes, *diced*
- 6 medium-sized potatoes, *diced*
- 1 small red onion, *quartered*
- 2 green peppers, *diced*
- 2 red bell peppers, *diced*
- 2 cups of onions, *finely chopped*
- 1/2 cup of olives, *pitted and sliced*
- 1/2 cup of raisins
- 1 teaspoon of garlic, *minced*
- 1 teaspoon of cumin, *ground*
- 1/2 teaspoon of cinnamon, *ground*
- 2 tablespoons of vinegar
- 1/2 teaspoon of sea salt
- 1/2 teaspoon of black pepper, *ground*
- 1/2 teaspoon of fennel seeds, *crushed*

- 2 cups of water

Direction:

- Combine the red onion quarters, green and red bell peppers, vinegar, and half the salt and oil in a plastic zipper bag.
- Seal the bag and shake to mix well.
- Heat the grill.
- In a large skillet, heat the rest of the oil.
- Add the chopped garlic and onion.
- Sauté for 5 minutes over medium heat.
- Add the cumin, cinnamon and fennel seeds and cook for another 2 minutes.
- Add the rest of the salt and 1/4th cup of water to the skillet.
- Add the olives, black pepper, tomatoes, raisins and potatoes, and bring to a boil.
- Reduce the heat and cover.
- Cook in low heat until the potatoes are tender.
- Discard the marinade from the pot.
- Remove the bell papers and the quartered onions from the plastic bag.
- Place all the vegetables on the grill.
- Grill for 15 minutes, turning the vegetables around frequently.

- Serve vegetables for a light lunch, or with couscous for a complete meal.

Servings: 4

Grilled Eggplant Sandwich

Ingredients:
- 2 large eggplants
- 1 Italian rye-bread, *cut into 8 small cubes*
- 2 cups of tomatoes, *cubed*
- 5 teaspoons of Parmesan cheese, *finely shredded*
- 1 cup of Mozzarella cheese, *shredded*
- 10 ounces of baby spinach
- 6 teaspoon of basil, *chopped*
- 6 teaspoon of olive oil, *extra virgin*
- 1/2 teaspoon of salt

Direction:
1. Preheat the grill.
2. Cut the eggplants into round slice of 1/2 inch thickness
3. Place the sliced eggplants on a baking tray.
4. Sprinkle salt on the eggplants.
5. Apply a coat of olive oil on both sides of the eggplants, and keep aside.

6. Put the spinach in a bowl and put inside the microwave.
7. Cover the bowl with a plastic sheet and make a few holes on it.
8. Microwave until the spinach wilts.
9. In another bowl, combine the tomatoes and half the basil.
10. Microwave until they start to bubble.
11. In a separate bowl, combine both the cheeses and keep aside.
12. Put all the ingredients together on the baking tray, with the eggplants.
13. Put the baking tray on the grill and cook until the eggplants are brown and soft.
14. Change sides 2/3 times until both sides are cooked.
15. Coat the bread cubes with olive oil on both sides.
16. Grill the bread until they are brown on both sides.
17. Layer the sandwiches - 1 piece of bread, 1 round of eggplant, 1 tablespoon of tomatoes and 1 teaspoon of cheese.
18. Repeat the process for all the ingredients until you have 8 individual sandwiches.

19. Put the sandwiches back on the grill and cook until the cheese melts.
20. Serve on 4 individual plates, 2 per each plate.

Servings: 4

Dinner

Lunches are quick affairs, but dinners are family oriented occasions when all your loved ones like to sit together and enjoy good food. Dinners in the Mediterranean diet are therefore, complex cuisines that the whole family can enjoy together.

Mediterranean-Style Fish Fillet

Ingredients:
- 2 pound of salmon fillet, cut into 8 pieces
- 4 tablespoons of white wine, dry
- 4 tablespoon of shallots, finely chopped
- 1/2 teaspoons of sea salt
- Lemon wedges, for garnish

Directions:

- Preheat your oven to 425°F.

- Coat an 8-inch baking dish with olive oil or cooking spray.
- Place the salmon fillets on the baking dish, skin side down.
- Sprinkle the wine on the fish fillets.
- Add the salt, pepper and shallots to the fillets.
- Cover the baking tray with foil and put it in the oven.
- Bake for 20 to 30 minutes, depending on how thick the fillets are.
- Transfer to 4 dinner plates, 2 on each.
- Sprinkle any leftover liquid from the baking pan on the fillets.
- Serve with lemon wedges for taste.

Servings: 4

Dinner Salad

A salad for dinner! Don't worry, there's plenty of vegetables in it to satisfy your appetite and keep you full.

Ingredients:

- 8 whole-wheat pitas, cut into wedges
- 4 cups of Romanian lettuce, shredded

- 1 cup of red onion, thinly sliced
- 1/2 cup of parsley, coarsely chopped
- 1 cups of feta cheese, crumbled
- 4 tablespoons of dill, coarsely chopped
- 4 cups of tomato, diced
- 1 tablespoon of capers
- 1 medium-sized cucumber, sliced
- 15 ounces of chickpeas (from a can), drained and dried
- 1 teaspoon of oregano, dried
- 2 tablespoons of lemon juice, freshly squeezed
- 2 tablespoons of olive oil, extra virgin

Direction:

- Combine together the parsley, dill and oregano with the olive oil and lemon juice.
- In a large salad bowl, add all the vegetables and beans together - the lettuce, tomatoes, cucumbers, capers, chickpeas and onions.
- Add the crumbled feta cheese.
- Toss well to mix.
- Serve with two pita breads per individual plate.

Servings: 4

Stuffed Tomatoes

We all love tomatoes as a part of our pizza, but here's a recipe where you can REALLY taste a good tomato!

Ingredients:

- 4 large tomatoes
- 1 cup of whole-grain croutons
- 1/2 cup of goat cheese, grated
- 1/2 cup of olives, pitted and halved
- 4 tablespoons of Italian salad dressing, low-fat or fat free
- 4 tablespoons of thyme, chopped

Direction:

- Preheat your broiler.
- Cut the top off the tomatoes.
- Use your fingers to pull out the seeds and the pulps from inside, leaving the shell.
- Drain the hollowed out tomatoes on a piece of paper.
- Chop the pulp pulled out from the tomatoes.

- In a large bowl, add the croutons, cheese, thyme, olives and dressing to the chopped tomato pulp.
- Mix well with a fork.
- Transfer the mixture to each of the hollowed out tomatoes.
- Put the tomatoes on a baking tray.
- Put the baking tray on the broiler and cook until the cheese melts.
- Serve hot.

Servings: 4

Chickpea Patties

By now, you must be craving for something a little spicy and fried! Perfect for the 4th day of this new diet - these chickpea patties would be great with pita bread or a salad on the side.

Ingredients:
- 15 ounces of chickpeas (from a can), rinsed and dried
- 1 clove of garlic, chopped
- 1/2 cup of parsley
- 1/2 teaspoon of cumin, ground

- 1/2 teaspoon of sea salt
- 1/2 teaspoon of black pepper
- 4 tablespoons of whole-grain flour
- 1 medium-sized egg, whisked
- 2 tablespoon of olive oil, extra virgin
- Extra virgin olive oil, for frying

Direction:

- In a food processor, blend together the parsley, cumin and garlic with the chickpeas until smooth.
- Add salt and pepper to the mixture and blend again.
- Transfer to a bowl.
- Add the egg to the mixture, and 2 half the whole-grain flour.
- Form into 8 individual patties with your hands, each 1/2 inch thick.
- Roll the patties on the remaining flour.
- Heat olive oil in a skillet over medium heat.
- Fry the patties in hot oil until golden brown.
- Serve with a salad, pita bread or yogurt.

Chicken Thighs Stuffed with Tomato Sauce

A chicken recipe that will make you forget you are on a diet and eating healthy.

Ingredients:

For the chicken and the stuffing

- 5 chicken thighs, *boneless and skinless, 5-ounce each*
- 1/2 cup of spinach, *cooked in water and drained*
- 2 ounces of chicken liver (optional), *chopped*
- 1/2 cup of whole-wheat breadcrumbs, *preferably day-old*
- 1/2 cup of Parmesan cheese, *freshly grated*
- 1 small egg, *whisked*
- 1 tablespoon of shallots, *chopped*
- 2 teaspoons of garlic, *minced*
- 1 teaspoon of thyme, *chopped*
- 1/2 teaspoon of pepper, *freshly ground*
- 1/4 teaspoon of salt
- 2 tablespoon of olive oil, *extra virgin*

For the Sauce

- 2 cups of broth, *preferably chicken*
- 1 cup of white wine, *dry*
- 30 ounces of tomatoes, *crushed*
- 1 cup of onion, *chopped*
- 1/2 cup of carrot, *finely chopped*
- 1/4 cup of shallots, *finely chopped*
- 1 tablespoon of garlic, *minced*
- 1 tablespoon of basil, *finely chopped*
- 1 teaspoon of thyme, *finely chopped*
- 1/4 teaspoon of pepper, *ground*
- A pinch of salt, *to taste*

Direction:

For the stuffed Chicken

- Combine the chicken livers (optional), breadcrumbs and spinach together in a large bowl.
- Add the parmesan cheese, shallots, egg, garlic, thyme, and the pepper and salt.
- Mix well.
- Cover and refrigerate for over 12 hours.
- Place the chicken thighs on a carving board and fill them up with the stuffing.
- Secure the stuffing inside the thighs with kitchen strings.

- Season with a pinch of salt and pepper.
- In a large skillet, heat oil over medium heat.
- Add the refrigerated chicken thighs on the oil.
- Cook for 15-20 minutes, turning over frequently, until the thighs are golden brown and cooked.
- Remove and keep aside.

For the sauce
- Heat 1 teaspoon of oil in a large skillet.
- Add the onion, garlic, carrot, shallots and fennel to the skillet.
- Cook until the vegetables are soft and cooked.
- Add the wine and bring to a boil.
- Cook for 10 minutes until the wine has reduced to half the amount.
- Add the broth, basil, thyme and tomatoes.
- Add the fried chicken thighs and bring to a boil.
- Reduce the heat and cook covered for at least 50 minutes.

- Frequently stir the chicken until they are cooked.
- Remove the thighs and keep covered in foil until dinnertime.
- Simmer the sauce to reduce to your desired thickness.
- Serve the chicken thighs on 5 individual plates, one in each plate.
- Top off with the sauce, as much as you prefer.

Servings: 5

Greek Pizza

Finally, a pizza for dinner that your whole family, especially your children, will love!
Ingredients:

- 1 whole wheat pizza dough, store bought
- 30 ounces of tomatoes, crushed by hand
- 2 cups of mozzarella cheese, fat free
- 1/2 cup of feta cheese, crumbled
- 1 cup of red pepper, roasted and cut into strips
- 1/2 cup of artichokes, marinated and halved

- 20 olives, pitted and halved
- 4 basil leaves, torn into pieces
- 1/2 teaspoon of oregano, dried

Direction:
- Preheat the oven to 500°F.
- Top the dough with hand-crushed tomatoes.
- Sprinkle dried oregano over the tomatoes.
- Spread the mozzarella cheese over the pizza dough.
- Distribute the rest of the toppings evenly on the cheese.
- Put the pizzas into the oven and bake until the cheese melts and the crust becomes golden brown.
- Remove pizza from the oven and sprinkle torn basil leaves.
- Cut the pizza into 8 slices and serve hot.

Servings: 4

Snacks

Snacking doesn't always have to be unhealthy processed foods. With the Mediterranean diet, your idea of snacks can also be healthy.

Olives-in-Herbs

The perfect snack to serve when you have friends over! Introduce them to the healthy Mediterranean lifestyle, too, and they will love it.

Ingredients:

- 2 cups of olives, canned or fresh
- 2 teaspoon of olive oil, extra-virgin
- 1 clove of garlic, crushed
- A pinch of oregano, dried
- A pinch of basil, dried
- A pinch of pepper, ground

Directions:

- Toss all the ingredients together.
- Serve fresh.

Servings: 12

Roasted Chickpeas

A great snack that you can munch on whenever hungry, or serve as a family snack during movie time, or at a party.

Ingredients:

- 2 cans of chickpeas, rinsed and pat dry
- Olive oil, for baking

- Sea salt and paprika, to taste

Directions:

- Line a baking tray with baking sheet.
- Lay down the dried chickpeas on it evenly.
- Drizzle olive oil on the chickpeas.
- Roast in an oven until the chickpeas become crunchy.
- Sprinkle some salt and pepper.
- Roast for 15 minutes more.
- Serve in a large bowl.

Servings: 4

Cream-covered Blueberries

Berries and cream, the perfect combination of a yummy snack or dessert that you'll love.

Ingredients:

- 4 cups of blueberries
- 8 ounces of low-fat cream
- 1.5 cups of yogurt, plain
- 4 teaspoons of lemon zest, freshly grated
- 2 tablespoon of honey

Direction:

- In a bowl, break the cream cheese with a fork.
- Add yogurt and honey to the cream cheese.
- Use an electric beater to mix the ingredients together into a smooth blend.
- Beat until the cream becomes light and foamy.
- Stir in the zest from the lemon.
- In individual desert dishes or glasses, layer in the blueberries.
- Pour in the lemon cream on top of the blueberries.

Servings: 4

Tomato Skewers

Everyone loves tomatoes, and they are going to love these delicious snacks made from tomatoes, mozzarella cheese and basil leaves.

Ingredients:

- 12 small mozzarella balls
- 12 cherry tomatoes
- 12 basil leaves
- 2 tablespoons of olive oil, extra virgin
- Sea salt and pepper, to taste

Direction:

- Use small skewers to thread mozzarella balls, tomatoes and basil leaves, one after another.
- Brush olive oil on all sides and sprinkle salt and pepper.
- In a big skillet over medium fire, fry the skewers for a few minutes until they start to turn a little dark.
  - Serve hot from the stove.

Servings: 3

Poached Pears

Finally, a snack that is also a dessert, but neither fattening nor bad for your health!

Ingredients:

- 8 pears, *whole*
- 2 cups of orange juice, *fresh*

- 1/2 cup of apple juice, *fresh*
- 1 cup of raspberries, *fresh*
- 2 teaspoons of nutmeg, *ground*
- 2 teaspoons of cinnamon, *ground*
- 4 tablespoons of orange zest, *freshly grated*

Directions:

- Combine the apple and orange juices in a bowl.
- Add the ground nutmeg and cinnamon.
- Stir well to mix.
- Peel the pears, but leave the stems behind.
- Remove the bottom part of the pears as well as the core.
- Place the pears in a wide, shallow pan.
- Pour in the juice.
- Cook in medium heat for at least half an hour.
- Turn the pears frequently.
  (Note: Let the liquid simmer but don't bring it to a boil.)
- Serve the pears in 4 individual dessert plates, 2 on each.

- Sprinkle orange zest on the pears.
  - Serve with fresh raspberries.

Servings: 4

Marinated Olives with Feta

Healthy olives marinated in spices and served with feta cheese - the perfect combination for a relaxed snack on a day off.

Ingredients:
- 2 cups of olives, *pitted and sliced*
- 1 cups of feta cheese, *diced*
- 1 teaspoon of rosemary, *chopped*
- Zest of 1 lemon, *freshly grated*
- Juice of 2 small lemons, *freshly squeezed*
- 4 cloves of garlic, *sliced*
- A pinch of black pepper, *crushed*
- Pepper to taste, *freshly ground*
- 4 tablespoons of olive oil, *extra virgin*

Direction:

- Combine all the ingredients together in a large bowl.

- Toss to mix well.
- Cover and put in the refrigerator for 24 hours.
- Serve cold.

Servings: 2

Mediterranean Rice Pudding

A dessert that is not too fattening and can be enjoyed guilt-free!

Ingredients:
- 1 cup of brown rice
- 6 cups of skim milk
- 2 tablespoons of honey
- 1/4 cup of raisins
- 1/2 teaspoon of cinnamon, *ground*
- 1/2 teaspoon of cardamom, *ground*
- 2 almonds, *finely chopped*
- 1/2 tablespoon of orange zest, *freshly grated*
- 1/2 teaspoon of rose water (optional)

Direction:

- Soak the rice in water for half an hour, then drain.

- In a large pan, pour in the milk.
- Add the honey and bring to a boil over medium-fire.
- Add the wet rice, the raisins and the cardamom and cinnamon to the milk.
- Cook in low heat for 50 minutes until the milk thickens.
- Stir frequently the whole time.
- Remove from heat.
- Sprinkle the rose water to the hot pudding.
- Pour the rice pudding into 4 individual dessert bowls.
- Combine the almond and orange zest and sprinkle over each bowl.
- Serve hot or cold, as preferred.

Servings: 4

These recipes were all wholesome, delicious, simple and very, very healthy for you and your family. Good luck in the kitchen when you try these recipes, because we guarantee that you will love them all!

Conclusion

This book was all about the Mediterranean diet - what the diet represents, how to adopt this diet into our lifestyles and what differences it can make to our health. Apart from the discussion on Mediterranean diet where you can learn everything there is to know about this diet, there is a complete list of what to eat and what not to eat that you will hopefully find very informative.

What is the most special feature of this book is a 7-day meal plan that you can easily establish in your lifestyle as well as in your family. This is a complete week-long meal plan that is balanced with the right amount of calories, carbohydrates and protein that your body needs, as well as the amount of serving per person.

Is it just the meal plan then? No! You will also find detailed recipes for each of the dishes mentioned in the meal plan - dishes that are easy, quick and delicious at the same time!

So what are you waiting for? Start your Mediterranean lifestyle right now, and stay healthy and happy forever!

Part 2

Introduction

I want to thank you and congratulate you for downloading the book, *"Mediterranean Diet"*.

This book contains how to lose weight by eating healthy.

The Mediterranean diet is, in fact, an amalgamation of aspects from the diets of several countries in the region. The basis for the diet boils down to the reduction of unhealthy fats, a decrease in the consumption of sweets and red meat, and an emphasis on fresh produce, fish and grains. The Mediterranean diet is designed as the antithesis of the American diet dominated by fat, sugar, and processed foods.

What is a Mediterranean Diet

The Mediterranean diet is, in fact, an amalgamation of aspects from the diets of several countries in the region. The basis for the diet boils down to the reduction of unhealthy fats, a decrease in the consumption of sweets and red meat, and an emphasis on fresh produce, fish, and grains. The Mediterranean diet is designed as the antithesis of the American diet dominated by fat, sugar, and processed foods.

Even though the Mediterranean diet is not of a specific country of origin, this mixed bag of nutritional guidelines can create a healthier heart, along with a number of other benefits associated with the a diet that does not rely heavily on junk food.

The Mediterranean diet draws from several regions including, Greece, Spain, and Italy. It is important to point out that not all aspects of the diet are shared with each country. Some of the countries that have inspired this diet do not adhere to some of its principles and vice versa. The Mediterranean diet is more of a collection of healthful dietary practices that have been in practice in the Mediterranean for centuries with promising results in the areas of illness and disease, and general health.

While most diet plans place an emphasis on the consumption of fresh food as opposed to processed foods and the like, the Mediterranean diet differs in its view of fats, salt, and protein. The Mediterranean diet is composed of moderate to liberal servings from the following categories:

Fish

Fruit

Vegetables

Legumes

Grains

Dairy

Unsaturated Fats

Wine

Meats

Fish make up a large portion of this diet plan. Salmon, tuna, mackerel, trout, and sardines are common sources of Omega-3 fatty acids, which promote brain health and help, defend against heart disease. Oysters and calamari are also sources of Omega-3. Foods known to prevent heart disease are a hallmark of the Mediterranean diet.

Fruits and vegetables rich in Vitamin C make up the bulk of the Mediterranean diet. Along with the low-fat, low calorie fish consumption, vegetables and fresh fruits are staples to the Greek diet, which the Mediterranean diet has adopted. Many times, snacks are often eaten in the form of varied produce, unlike American snacks which consist of processed foods high in salt content and swimming in high fructose corn syrup and saturated fats.

Legumes, or beans, lentils, chickpeas, and the like, are healthy and filling options allowed in the Mediterranean diet. Grains are often consumed in the form of whole grain breads, polenta, couscous, and pasta. Another departure from American eating habits, bread consumed in the Mediterranean is usually dipped in olive oil, either plain or flavored with herbs or garlic. It is more common in America for bread to be slathered with butter, which is forbidden on the Mediterranean diet. Olive and canola oils act as a substitute for butter.

Dairy products are consumed with this diet but on a much smaller scale that seafood and produce. The dairy eaten is mostly in the form of milk, fresh cheese, and yogurt.

Olive oil is the cornerstone of the Mediterranean diet. Olive oil replaces traditionally used fats in favor of its more healthful components. Known as a "good fat", olive oil has been found to increase good cholesterol in the blood and lower the risk for heart disease and other common ailments.

The Mediterranean and parts of Europe are associated with wine consumption with meals more frequently than Americans and those from northern European nations. Though somewhat controversial, there are studies touting the benefits of moderate red wine consumption. This is due to red wine's antioxidant properties, making wine a healthier choice than beer, carbonated beverages, and sugary fruit juices combined.

Other forms of protein are not forbidden under the Mediterranean diet plan, but they are restricted. Skinless, white meat chicken and turkey, would be the best go-to options for this diet, but very occasional meals featuring red meat is not condemned. American diets rely heavily on red meat, but this can be detrimental to heart health. By reducing red meat intake, a person's overall health can improve dramatically.

Salty foods are also a staple of the Mediterranean diet. Olives, capers, anchovies, and other cured delicacies are commonplace in Mediterranean cuisine, and should be eaten in moderation. On the upside, because of the high salt content of many on the foods in this plan, adding salt to food is unwarranted.

Nuts are another snack option that should be approached with a light hand. Nuts are naturally loaded with fat, but the fat is the "good" kind. Nevertheless, nuts should only be a small snack, not a robust one.

The Mediterranean diet differs in comparison to traditional diet plans by placing significance on fat intake. Only the fat for this diet is good for the body. The flavorful and varied menu of the Mediterranean diet eases the sting of being on a diet. In fact, the diet allows a person to enjoy their meals instead of dreading them, making this diet a pleasant experience to be incorporated into one's lifestyle on a permanent basis rather than a test of endurance with a much coveted end date.

What Foods are Included in the Mediterranean Diet

In general, the Mediterranean diet is comprised of fresh, healthful ingredients. The majority of foods allowed via the diet are produce, fresh fish, and grains. Processed foods and foods rife with chemically enhanced ingredients and fillers are entirely off the menu. That is not to say that fat salt are absent from the diet, however. Many foods are naturally salty or fatty. The Mediterranean diet takes advantage of this tendency, encouraging the consumption of "good" fats, naturally occurring sugars, and foods that are salty in their own right, rather than by an overly liberal hand.

This section breaks down foods by categories and lists the best food options for an individual following the Mediterranean diet.

Fish

Fish, as a protein, should be the number one choice for someone on the Mediterranean diet. A valuable source of omega-3 fatty acids, fish is naturally low in fat, comes in an incredible variety of options, and is versatile in both methods of cooking and seasoning.

Eating fish several times a week in place of red meats is a healthier, smarter choice for those looking to improve overall health and lose weight. It should be noted that this category is not limited to strictly fish. Many seafood choices can provide the same vitamins, minerals, and omega-3 benefits as fish, but on a broader spectrum of choice.

The following are just a few of the fish and seafood options available to Mediterranean dieters:

Anchovies

Cod

Clams

Crab

Halibut

Lobster

Mackerel

Mussels

Salmon

Sardines

Scallops

Sea Bass

Shrimp

Squid

Trout

Tuna

Whiting

Fruit

One of the biggest failings of the classic American and northern European diet is the affinity for sweets. Though people with a nagging sweet tooth may find it difficult, nee impossible to replace cakes, cookies, and candy with fruit, it is worth the effort to cut down as much as possible. Fresh fruit, in many instances has natural sugars, making them sweet tasting. This can certainly satisfy a craving for sweets, especially if the Mediterranean diet is taken seriously as a lifestyle change.

Eating fresh fruit for a dessert may take some getting used to, especially for those so unaccustomed to this type healthy eating, but the health benefits far outweigh the craving for the cloying sweetness of added sugar and sweeteners that traditional American desserts are often composed of.

Fresh produce are an essential part to the Mediterranean diet. Replacing unhealthy snacks, junk food, and sweets with fresh, vitamin-packed options, cuts down on calories, fat intake, and harmful added chemicals and preservatives.

A few examples of fruits include:

Apples

Bananas

Cherries

Figs

Grapes

Mangoes

Melons

Olives

Oranges

Pears

Pineapples

Plums

Tomatoes

Vegetables

Fresh fruits and vegetables contain antioxidant properties that ward off illness. Eating an abundance of fresh produce only increases the immune system's ability to function well and build up the defenses in a body.

Many people complain about disliking certain vegetables, either because of taste or texture, but there exist a myriad of produce options that can be sampled, experimented with, and perfected. Simply because a diet plan lists certain foods as acceptable, does not mean that all the foods are required to be eaten. A good rule of thumb is to try everything at least once, and determine what is to your taste.

Keep in mind that the simpler the preparation, the more healthful the food will be. Masking foods in an overabundance of salt, gravy, dip, or sauce just adds calories, sodium, and fat, canceling out the benefits of eating the vegetable altogether.

A condensed list of vegetables on the Mediterranean diet plan includes:

Asparagus

Bean Sprouts

Beets

Broccoli

- Brussels Sprouts
- Cabbage
- Carrots
- Cauliflower
- Celery
- Chili Peppers
- Collard Greens
- Cucumbers
- Eggplant
- Fennel
- Garlic
- Green Beans
- Jicama
- Leeks
- Lettuce
- Mushrooms
- Onions
- Parsnips

Peppers

Shallots

Spinach

Yellow Squash

Zucchini

Legumes

Legumes are essentially plants grown in pods. There is a wide variety of this type of plant, and, very often legumes are not associated with one another as being the same type of food. Legumes are sources of fiber and protein, and can act as a substitute for less healthy options with meals.

Legumes range from shelled beans to entirely edible pod casings. Fresh, dried, or frozen legumes would be the healthiest choices. Canned beans often contain sauces or gravies, or are loaded with salt for flavor and preservation purposes. Stick with the more natural offerings.

Choices of legumes include the following:

Black Beans

Black Eyed Peas

Cannellini Beans

Chick Peas

Cranberry Beans

Edamame

Great Northern Beans

Green Peas

Kidney Beans

Lentils

Lima Beans

Navy Beans

Okra

Peanuts

Pinto Beans

Snow Peas

Sugar Snap Peas

Grains

Incorporating whole grains into a diet can be as easy as switching from white bread to eating breads made from whole grains. However, for people accustomed to eating white bread or white rice, the change may require an adjustment to their mindset. Not only are whole grains healthier, but products such as bread made from whole grain using less sugar than their white bread counterparts. The additional fiber content that comes with whole grains products is another bonus.

Grains can also be served as accompaniments with meals. Replacing starches with little dietary value with a whole grain can make the difference between eating foods that are nearly empty calories and eating foods that improve health and the functions of the body.

Some of the most common grains available are:

Barley

Brown Rice

Corn

Wheat

Dairy

Calcium is important to strengthen bones and teeth, but the downside is that dairy products usually contain exorbitant amounts of fat. The Mediterranean diet allows limited servings of dairy, mostly in the form of fresh cheeses or yogurt. Eaten in moderation, dairy is good occasional snack option, but one that should never be overindulged. Low fat and non-fat dairy products are smart choices when eating dairy. Note that ice cream is not included due to added sugar and a high fat content.

Dairy, in its many forms, can include:

Blue Cheese

Buttermilk

Cheddar Cheese

Cottage Cheese

Cream Cheese

Feta Cheese

Goat Cheese

Mozzarella Cheese

Parmesan Cheese

Romano Cheese

Ricotta Cheese

Milk

Sour Cream

Yogurt

Unsaturated Fats

Saturated fats raise cholesterol levels, clog arteries, and increase blood pressure. As a general rule, saturated fat should be avoided at every turn. Unfortunately, due to the overuse of butter in American cuisine, this is rarely the case. Mediterranean diets, though not all, rely heavily on the use of olive oil to replace the dangerous fat content of butter and other oils used for cooking, or as accompaniments.

Olive oil, as well as a few other sources, contains unsaturated fats. These fats increase LDL cholesterol levels, which are good for humans. By substituting "good" fat for the harmful variety, an individual can eliminate saturated fats as a factor for elevated bad cholesterol levels and a risk of heart disease.

Unsaturated fats can be found in the following:

Avocados

Canola Oil

Grapeseed Oil

Olive Oil

Wine

Though still controversial, there have been an increasing numbers of scientific studies in recent years that have touted the positive health effects of drinking red wine. Moderate consumption of red wine has been linked to a decreased risk of heart disease. It should be noted that people with a personal or family history of alcoholism should not partake of this particular suggestion, as it is optional, but for those willing and able to adhere to this part of the Mediterranean diet, it can be potentially beneficial.

Meats

An all fish diet, especially in the case of the American palate, is not likely to be appealing. However, there are other proteins that make good alternatives throughout the week. Poultry and pork options can be just as healthful as fish as long as certain measures are taken to ensure that the meat is stripped of its unfavorable trappings. Namely, skin and fat.

Poultry should be skinless, and any meat should be meticulously trimmed of fat, to create the leanest cut of meat possible. Fat used for cooked, if needed, should consist of an unsaturated fat listed in the category above.

Alternative proteins include:

Chicken

Pork

Turkey

Nuts and Seeds

Nuts and seeds can be a wonderful, healthy alternative to traditional snacks. Instead of reaching for heavily salted potato chips or a pre-packaged box of cookies, a handful of roasted nuts or seeds can easily assuage an appetite between meals.

A word of caution is on order, though. Nuts are naturally high in fat and can quickly add up in calories because of this. The fat is usually the healthful kind, but these treats should be eaten sparsely for those seeking to lose weight. Also, be wary of salted and flavored nut and seed varieties. Many of those contain extreme amounts of sodium, which defeats the purpose of choosing nuts and seeds in the first place.

Some seeds and nuts that can be found include:

Almonds

Brazil Nuts

Cashews

Chestnuts

Poppy Seeds

Pumpkin Seeds

Sesame Seeds

Sunflower Seeds

Walnuts

What Not To Eat

Under the Mediterranean diet, foods that offer little of no nutritional value are either forbidden or drastically restricted. For an American, this could mean a big change in eating habits. Butter, processed foods, and most sweets are virtually eliminated. The same can be said for adding salt to food. As many foods under the plan are naturally salty, this should make that rule easier to stick with.

Red meat and eggs are other severely limited foods. Red meat can lead to heart disease, and digestive problems, and dieters are discouraged from eating beef, lamb, and game, if not entirely, then only a few times a month. Eggs are also nearly absent from the Mediterranean diet. Eggs are a source of protein, but can also raise cholesterol, resulting in the egg playing a reduced role in the Mediterranean diet in comparison to a traditional American eating habit.

Processed foods, along with packaged snacks and foods also include bacon, sausage, and hot dogs. All are highly processed meats with little dietary value.

Restricted foods include:

Butter

Eggs

Red Meat

Processed Foods

Sweets

Additional Salt

All restricted foods can be replaced with healthier options. Olive oil can replace butter in most instances. Fish and poultry can fill the void left by red meat, and salting food can be avoided by seasoning foods with herbs and spices, or by eating foods that are already salt and require no further seasoning.

The biggest change may very well be eliminating processed foods and sweets from your diet. This could take time getting used to but the health benefits are worth the period of adjustment.

What are the Health Benefits of the Mediterranean Diet

There is a number of positive health effects associated with the Mediterranean diet. Because the diet cuts out most saturated fats in favor of monounsaturated fat, cardiovascular risk factors are greatly reduced. Cholesterol and blood pressures can be reduced, and heart disease risks diminished.

Cutting out processed foods, sugary foods, and red meat also plays a significant role in the heart disease risk reduction, as well as lowering the chances of developing diabetes, or brain related ailments like Alzheimer's.

How to Lose Weight on the Mediterranean Diet

As with most diets, portion control is key to losing weight. Because the Mediterranean diet is loaded with healthy fat, that means calories can quickly add up. Keeping portions small and choosing what you eat and when wisely will go a long way to achieving a weight loss goal.

In addition to controlling fat intake, it would also be smart to begin taking supplements containing iron and calcium to bolster the immune system and make up for the absence of red meat and the reduction of dairy consumption.

Implementing a Mediterranean Diet Plan

Here are some helpful hints to sticking with the diet successfully:

Choose fresh produce and fish

Switch to whole grain bread, pasta, rice, and cereal

Snack on fresh fruit and vegetables

Ban butter from the refrigerator

Flavor food with fresh herbs and dried spices

Choose low-fat options

Sample Meal Plan

Breakfast

Sliced honeydew melon

Whole wheat toast

½ cup Greek yogurt

Lunch

Baked chicken breast

Brown rice

Edamame

Snacks

Baby carrots

Roasted sunflower seeds

Dinner

Cod with Tomatoes and Olives

Spinach salad

Recipe

Ingredients:

4 Cod Fillets

1/4 teaspoon freshly ground black pepper

1 1/2 tablespoons extra-virgin olive oil

1 yellow onion, finely chopped

2 cloves garlic, minced

3 tomatoes, diced

½ cup green olives, sliced

1 tablespoon capers

2 tablespoons lime juice

Directions:

Heat 1 tablespoon of the olive oil in a skillet. Season the fish with pepper and add to the pan, searing both sides for 2-3 minutes. Remove from skillet and keep warm. Add remaining olive oil to skillet. Sauté onions until soft. Add garlic and cook 1 minute. Add remaining ingredients except lime juice. Simmer 15 minutes. Return cod to the skillet and finish cooking the fish. Add lime juice and serve with a spinach salad topped with sliced, toasted almonds and sliced cucumbers, and dressed with olive oil and lemon juice.

Dessert

Fruit salad with apples, grapes, oranges, and pineapple

Conclusion

It is my sincere hope that you might have liked all the recipes which have been mentioned in the book and once again thank you for getting this book and experimenting with the recipes.

About The Author

Ernest Valentine is born with the vision to promote *Mediterranean diet* among the masses. The author has written several research papers on the topic. He has served as an instructor promoting various cultural arts in University of San Francisco. He is currently living with his spouse in Texas.

www.ingramcontent.com/pod-product-compliance
Lightning Source LLC
LaVergne TN
LVHW011956070526
838202LV00054B/4935